LECTIN-FREE DIET COOKBOOK AND FOODLIST FOR ADULTS

The Ultimate Guide to Achieve Weight Loss, Fight Inflammation and Improve Gut Health with Easy, Delicious and Nutritious Recipes.

Olivia Endwell

Copyright Statement:

Disclaimer:

The information provided in this book is for educational and informational purposes only. It is not intended as a substitute for professional medical advice, diagnosis, or treatment. Always seek the advice of your physician or other qualified health provider with any questions you may have regarding a medical condition. Never disregard professional medical advice or delay in seeking it because of something you have read in this book.

The author and publisher disclaim any liability arising directly or indirectly from the use of this book. The information provided is based on the author's best knowledge at the time of writing and is subject to change. The author and publisher do not guarantee the accuracy, completeness, or timeliness of the information presented in this book.

Individual results may vary, and the success of any dietary or lifestyle change depends on various factors, including but not limited to individual commitment and adherence. Before making significant changes to your diet or lifestyle, consult with a qualified healthcare professional.

The views and opinions expressed in this book are those of the author and do not necessarily reflect the official policy or position of any other agency, organization, employer, or company.

TABLE OF CONTENTS

INTRODUCTION

Embarking on a journey toward a lectin-free lifestyle involves a profound understanding of the dietary choices we make and their impact on our well-being. In this introduction, we will delve into the intricacies of lectins, shedding light on their role in our diet and the potential effects they may have on our health. Through a comprehensive exploration, we aim to equip you with the knowledge needed to make informed decisions about what goes onto your plate.

As we navigate the realms of nutrition, the spotlight will illuminate the compelling benefits that a lectin-free diet can offer. From enhanced digestive health to potential alleviation of inflammation, we will uncover the science behind these advantages, providing you with a compelling rationale to embrace a lectin-free approach to eating.

Moreover, the question arises – who stands to gain the most from adopting a lectin-free diet? We will unravel the demographics and conditions that may find solace in this dietary shift. Whether you're grappling with specific health concerns or simply seeking a proactive approach to well-being, the insights provided will help you ascertain if a lectin-free lifestyle aligns with your personal goals and aspirations.

In the pages that follow, we invite you to embark on a journey of discovery, empowerment, and holistic well-being. Together, we'll navigate the intricate tapestry of lectins, unraveling the benefits that a lectin-free diet can offer, and identifying who can reap the rewards of this transformative dietary path.

CHAPTER 1: GETTING STARTED WITH THE LECTIN-FREE DIET

Assessing Your Current Diet

Embarking on the journey of adopting a lectin-free diet begins with a thoughtful examination of your current eating habits. This introspective process serves as a crucial foundation, allowing you to identify patterns, assess nutritional imbalances, and recognize the presence of lectin-rich foods in your daily meals.

Start by keeping a detailed food journal for a week. Record everything you eat, including snacks, beverages, and condiments. Take note of portion sizes and the frequency of certain foods. This exercise serves as an eye-opener, revealing not only what you consume but also highlighting potential triggers for discomfort or inflammation.

As you scrutinize your food journal, pay special attention to foods known to contain lectins. These include grains, legumes, certain nightshades, and processed foods. Consider how these items feature in your diet and whether they coincide with any digestive issues or unexplained discomfort you may be experiencing. This reflective process sets the stage for a mindful transition to a lectin-free lifestyle.

Beyond mere observation, it's crucial to evaluate the nutritional aspects of your current diet. Are you obtaining a balanced intake of essential nutrients? Assess the diversity of fruits, vegetables, proteins, and fats in your meals. This evaluation helps you understand the potential nutritional gaps in your current diet, guiding the formulation of a lectin-free eating plan that ensures optimal nourishment.

By taking the time to assess your current diet, you lay the groundwork for a personalized and effective lectin-free journey. Armed with insights into your dietary habits and their impact, you are better equipped to make informed choices and transition toward a lectin-free lifestyle that aligns with your health goals.

Foods to Avoid

Navigating the terrain of a lectin-free diet involves a keen awareness of foods to avoid, as lectin-containing items can contribute to various health issues. Understanding which foods harbor lectins empowers you to make intentional choices that align with your dietary goals and overall well-being.

Grains: Grains, such as wheat, barley, and rye, are notorious for their lectin content. Found in many staple foods like bread and pasta, these grains can be a significant source of lectins in the diet. Transitioning to lectin-free alternatives like almond flour or coconut flour opens up a world of possibilities for creating delicious, grain-free meals.

Legumes: Beans, lentils, and peanuts are rich in lectins, making them prime candidates for exclusion in a lectin-free diet. While these foods are often celebrated for their protein and fiber content, lectins can interfere with digestion and nutrient absorption. Exploring alternative protein sources, such as lean meats and seafood, becomes essential for maintaining a balanced diet.

Nightshades: Certain vegetables from the nightshade family, including tomatoes, eggplants, and bell peppers, contain lectins that may pose challenges for some individuals. While these vegetables offer valuable nutrients, those on a lectin-free journey may need to experiment with excluding or limiting nightshades to observe their impact on personal health.

Processed Foods: Processed and packaged foods often hide lectins in various forms. From preservatives to additives, these substances can undermine your efforts to maintain a lectin-free diet. Reading labels attentively and opting for whole, unprocessed foods ensures you steer clear of hidden lectin sources while embracing nutrient-dense alternatives.

By being mindful of these common sources of lectins, you pave the way for a lectin-free diet that supports your health goals. Experimenting with creative substitutes and diversifying your plate with lectin-free options allows you to savor delicious meals while prioritizing your well-being.

Foods to Embrace

Transitioning to a lectin-free diet opens the door to a vibrant array of nutrient-dense foods that nourish your body and contribute to overall wellness. Embracing lectin-free alternatives empowers you to craft delicious, satisfying meals while reaping the benefits of a diet that supports optimal digestion and health.

Leafy Greens: Leafy greens, such as kale, spinach, and Swiss chard, stand out as nutritional powerhouses in a lectin-free diet. Rich in vitamins, minerals, and antioxidants, these greens contribute to overall well-being while offering versatility in salads, smoothies, and cooked dishes.

Cruciferous Vegetables: Broccoli, cauliflower, and Brussels sprouts are excellent choices for a lectin-free diet. These cruciferous vegetables not only provide essential nutrients but also add delightful flavors and textures to your meals. Roasting or sautéing them with healthy fats enhances both taste and nutritional value.

Berries: Antioxidant-rich berries, including blueberries, strawberries, and raspberries, are sweet indulgences in a lectin-free diet. Packed with vitamins and fiber, these fruits make for satisfying snacks or additions to breakfast options like lectin-free smoothies or yogurt alternatives.

Healthy Fats: Avocado, olive oil, and fatty fish offer valuable sources of healthy fats in a lectin-free eating plan. These fats not only contribute to satiety but also support cognitive function and heart health. Incorporating them into your meals ensures a well-rounded and flavorful approach to lectin-free living.

Lean Proteins: As you navigate away from lectin-rich legumes, lean proteins become essential components of your lectin-free diet. Options such as poultry, fish, and grass-fed meats supply the protein necessary for muscle health and overall vitality.

By embracing these lectin-free alternatives, you not only create a diverse and satisfying menu but also provide your body with the nutrients it needs to thrive. Experimenting with new recipes and enjoying the variety of lectin-free foods available ensures that your journey towards a lectin-free lifestyle is both delicious and enriching.

CHAPTER 3: THE LECTIN-FREE KITCHEN

Stocking Your Pantry

Creating a lectin-free kitchen begins with thoughtful and strategic stocking of your pantry. The key is to replace lectin-rich items with nutritious alternatives, ensuring that your culinary creations align with your lectin-free goals while maintaining a diverse and satisfying diet.

Flour Alternatives: Traditional flours like wheat and all-purpose flour are laden with lectins. Transitioning to lectin-free alternatives such as almond flour, coconut flour, or cassava flour opens up a world of possibilities for baking and cooking. These alternatives not only serve as effective substitutes but also bring unique flavors and textures to your dishes.

Grains and Legume Replacements: Bid farewell to lectin-heavy grains and legumes by introducing lectin-free alternatives into your pantry. Quinoa, millet, and lentils without the lectin-rich outer coating can be excellent substitutes. Experimenting with these alternatives allows you to maintain the texture and nutritional benefits of traditional grains and legumes without compromising your lectin-free commitment.

Canned Goods: Many canned goods, including beans and tomatoes, are common sources of lectins. Opt for lectin-free alternatives like canned coconut milk, artichoke hearts, and water-packed tuna. These choices not only align with a lectin-free lifestyle but also contribute to the variety of flavors you can incorporate into your meals.

Sauces and Condiments: Traditional sauces and condiments often harbor hidden lectins. Explore lectin-free alternatives such as homemade dressings with olive oil and lemon, tomato-free marinara sauces, and coconut aminos instead of soy sauce. Building a repertoire of lectin-free condiments ensures that your meals are not only flavorful but also free from potential lectin pitfalls.

Nuts and Seeds: While nuts and seeds are generally lectin-free, it's essential to be mindful of portion sizes. Incorporate lectin-free varieties like almonds, chia seeds, and flaxseeds into your pantry for a nutrient-rich boost to salads, smoothies, or as snacks. These items not only provide essential nutrients but also contribute to the satisfying textures of your meals.

By strategically curating your pantry with lectin-free alternatives, you set the stage for a kitchen that supports your journey towards optimal health. This intentional approach ensures that every ingredient contributes to the flavor, texture, and nutritional profile of your lectin-free meals.

Essential Kitchen Tools

Equipping your kitchen with the right tools is a fundamental step towards mastering the art of lectin-free cooking. These essential items not only make your cooking process more efficient but also enable you to explore a variety of techniques that enhance the flavor and texture of lectin-free dishes.

High-Quality Blender: A powerful blender is a must-have in a lectin-free kitchen. It opens up a world of possibilities for creating smoothies, sauces, and soups without the need for lectin-rich ingredients. Invest in a blender that can handle tough ingredients like fibrous vegetables and frozen fruits, ensuring that your lectin-free creations are both delicious and convenient.

Food Processor: A food processor is a versatile tool that simplifies the preparation of lectin-free meals. From finely chopping vegetables to creating lectin-free nut-based flours, this kitchen essential streamlines the cooking process. Look for a durable and multi-functional food processor that can handle a variety of tasks.

Spiralizer: For pasta lovers on a lectin-free journey, a spiralizer is a game-changer. This tool transforms vegetables like zucchini and sweet potatoes into noodle-like strands, providing a lectin-free alternative to traditional pasta. Experiment with different vegetables to discover your favorite lectin-free noodle substitutes.

Cast Iron Skillet: A cast iron skillet is a staple in lectin-free cooking. It not only enhances the flavor of your dishes but also provides an excellent non-stick surface without the need for harmful coatings. From sautéing vegetables to searing proteins, a cast iron skillet is a versatile and durable addition to your kitchen arsenal.

Quality Knives: Investing in high-quality knives is essential for efficient and precise food preparation. From chopping vegetables to deboning meats, a sharp set of knives ensures that you can navigate the variety of lectin-free ingredients with ease. Regular sharpening and proper care are crucial to maintaining the longevity of your knives.

By outfitting your kitchen with these essential tools, you empower yourself to explore the full spectrum of lectin-free cooking techniques. These tools not only enhance the efficiency of your kitchen but also open up a world of culinary possibilities, allowing you to savor the creativity and diversity of lectin-free meals.

Cooking Techniques for a Lectin-Free Lifestyle

Mastering cooking techniques tailored to a lectin-free lifestyle is the key to creating flavorful and satisfying meals. Whether you're a seasoned chef or a novice in the kitchen, embracing these techniques ensures that your lectin-free dishes are not only nutritious but also a delight to the senses.

Sautéing and Stir-Frying: Sautéing and stir-frying are quick and versatile techniques that allow you to cook vegetables and proteins without compromising their lectin-free status. Use lectin-free oils like olive oil or avocado oil to impart delicious flavors while preserving the nutritional integrity of your ingredients.

Roasting and Baking: Roasting and baking are ideal techniques for bringing out the natural sweetness and flavors of vegetables and proteins. Use your oven to create lectin-free roasted vegetables, chicken, or fish. Experiment with herbs and spices to add depth to your dishes without relying on lectin-rich seasonings.

Steaming: Steaming is a gentle cooking method that retains the nutritional value of vegetables while imparting a crisp and vibrant texture. Invest in a quality steamer to prepare lectin-free broccoli, cauliflower, and other vegetables. Steaming is particularly effective for preserving the color and crunchiness of your ingredients.

Grilling: Grilling is a fantastic way to add a smoky flavor to your lectin-free dishes. Choose lectin-free proteins like grass-fed meats, poultry, or fish and grill them to perfection. Pairing grilled items with lectin-free marinades or herb-infused oils enhances the overall taste and appeal.

Raw Preparations: Embracing raw preparations, such as salads and ceviche, is a refreshing approach to lectin-free cooking. Incorporate a variety of colorful vegetables, fruits, and lean proteins to create vibrant and nutrient-packed meals. Raw preparations are not only visually appealing but also offer a delightful contrast in textures.

Fermentation: Fermentation is a technique that adds depth of flavor and promotes gut health in a lectin-free diet. Explore lacto-fermented vegetables like sauerkraut or kimchi, which not only serve as flavorful condiments but also contribute to a healthy gut microbiome. Homemade fermented foods allow you to tailor the flavors to your liking while ensuring lectin-free compliance.

As you experiment with these cooking techniques, you'll discover a world of possibilities within the realm of lectin-free cuisine. Embrace the creativity and flexibility that lectin-free cooking offers, allowing you to enjoy delicious and nutritious meals that align with your health goals. With these techniques at your disposal, your journey towards a lectin-free lifestyle becomes a culinary adventure filled with flavor and vitality.

CHAPTER 3: BREAKFAST RECIPES

1. Lectin-Free Berry Smoothie Bowl

Prep Time: 10 minutes

Cooking Time: 0 minutes

Serving Size: 1

Ingredients:

- 1 cup mixed berries (strawberries, blueberries, raspberries)
- 1/2 ripe avocado
- 1/2 cup unsweetened almond milk
- 1 tablespoon chia seeds
- 1 tablespoon almond butter
- Ice cubes (optional)
- Fresh mint leaves for garnish

Instructions:

1. In a blender, combine the mixed berries, ripe avocado, almond milk, chia seeds, and almond butter.
2. Blend until smooth and creamy. Add ice cubes if you prefer a colder consistency.

3. Pour the smoothie into a bowl.

4. Garnish with fresh mint leaves.

5. Enjoy your lectin-free berry smoothie bowl!

Nutritional Information:

- Calories: 350

- Protein: 7g

- Carbohydrates: 30g

- Fiber: 12g

- Sugars: 12g

- Fat: 25g

- Saturated Fat: 3g

- Sodium: 80mg

2. Spinach and Tomato Omelette

Prep Time: 5 minutes

Cooking Time: 10 minutes

Serving Size: 2

Ingredients:

- 4 large eggs

- 1 cup fresh spinach, chopped

- 1/2 cup cherry tomatoes, halved

- 1/4 cup red onion, finely chopped

- 2 tablespoons olive oil

- Salt and pepper to taste

Instructions:

1. In a bowl, whisk the eggs until well beaten. Season with salt and pepper.

2. Heat olive oil in a non-stick skillet over medium heat.

3. Add chopped spinach, cherry tomatoes, and red onion to the skillet. Sauté until the vegetables are tender.

4. Pour the beaten eggs over the vegetables, ensuring an even distribution.

5. Cook until the edges set, then gently lift and fold the omelette.

6. Continue cooking until the eggs are fully set.

7. Serve hot.

Nutritional Information:

- Calories: 280

- Protein: 14g

- Carbohydrates: 6g

- Fiber: 2g

- Sugars: 3g

- Fat: 22g

- Saturated Fat: 5g

- Sodium: 220mg

3. Almond Flour Pancakes

Prep Time: 10 minutes

Cooking Time: 15 minutes

Serving Size: 4 pancakes

Ingredients:

- 1 cup almond flour

- 2 large eggs

- 1/2 cup almond milk

- 1 tablespoon coconut oil, melted

- 1 teaspoon baking powder

- 1/2 teaspoon vanilla extract

- Pinch of salt

Instructions:

1. In a bowl, whisk together almond flour, baking powder, and salt.

2. In a separate bowl, beat eggs and add almond milk, melted coconut oil, and vanilla extract. Mix well.

3. Combine wet and dry ingredients, stirring until a smooth batter forms.

4. Heat a griddle or non-stick skillet over medium heat.

5. Pour 1/4 cup of batter for each pancake onto the griddle.

6. Cook until bubbles form on the surface, then flip and cook the other side until golden brown.

7. Repeat with the remaining batter.

8. Serve warm with your favorite lectin-free toppings.

Nutritional Information:

- Calories: 220

- Protein: 8g

- Carbohydrates: 7g

- Fiber: 3g

- Sugars: 1g

- Fat: 18g

- Saturated Fat: 3g

- Sodium: 280mg

4. Avocado and Smoked Salmon Breakfast Wrap

Prep Time: 15 minutes
Cooking Time: 0 minutes
Serving Size: 1

Ingredients:

- 1 large collard green leaf (used as a wrap)

- 1/2 ripe avocado, sliced

- 2 ounces smoked salmon

- 1/4 cup cucumber, julienned

- 1 tablespoon capers

- Fresh dill for garnish

Instructions:

1. Lay the collard green leaf flat on a clean surface.

2. Arrange avocado slices, smoked salmon, cucumber, and capers in the center of the leaf.

3. Carefully fold the sides of the leaf and then roll it tightly, creating a wrap.

4. Slice in half and secure with toothpicks if needed.

5. Garnish with fresh dill.

6. Enjoy your lectin-free avocado and smoked salmon wrap!

Nutritional Information:

- Calories: 320

- Protein: 15g

- Carbohydrates: 12g

- Fiber: 8g

- Sugars: 1g

- Fat: 25g

- Saturated Fat: 4g

- Sodium: 780mg

5. Chia Seed Pudding Parfait

Prep Time: 5 minutes (plus overnight chilling)
Cooking Time: 0 minutes
Serving Size: 1

Ingredients:

- 2 tablespoons chia seeds

- 1/2 cup unsweetened almond milk

- 1/4 teaspoon vanilla extract

- 1/2 cup mixed berries (blueberries, raspberries, strawberries)

- 1 tablespoon unsweetened coconut flakes

Instructions:

1. In a bowl, mix chia seeds, almond milk, and vanilla extract. Stir well.

2. Cover the bowl and refrigerate overnight or for at least 4 hours until the chia seeds have absorbed the liquid and formed a pudding-like consistency.

3. In a glass or jar, layer the chia seed pudding with mixed berries.

4. Repeat the layers.

5. Top with coconut flakes.

6. Enjoy your lectin-free chia seed pudding parfait!

Nutritional Information:

- Calories: 280

- Protein: 8g

- Carbohydrates: 26g

- Fiber: 12g

- Sugars: 8g

- Fat: 18g

- Saturated Fat: 6g

- Sodium: 100mg

6. Sweet Potato and Kale Breakfast Hash

Prep Time: 15 minutes

Cooking Time: 20 minutes

Serving Size: 2

Ingredients:

- 2 medium sweet potatoes, peeled and diced

- 1 cup kale, chopped

- 1/2 red bell pepper, diced

- 1/4 cup red onion, finely chopped

- 2 tablespoons olive oil

- 4 large eggs

- Salt and pepper to taste

Instructions:

1. In a skillet, heat olive oil over medium heat.

2. Add diced sweet potatoes and sauté until golden brown and cooked through.

3. Add chopped kale, red bell pepper, and red onion. Cook until vegetables are tender.

4. Make four wells in the hash and crack an egg into each well.

5. Cover the skillet and cook until the eggs are cooked to your liking.

6. Season with salt and pepper.

7. Serve hot.

Nutritional Information:

- Calories: 380

- Protein: 12g

- Carbohydrates: 32g

- Fiber: 6g

- Sugars: 8g

- Fat: 24g

- Saturated Fat: 5g

- Sodium: 220mg

7. Coconut Flour Crepes with Berries

Prep Time: 10 minutes

Cooking Time: 10 minutes

Serving Size: 2

Ingredients:

- 1/2 cup coconut flour

- 4 large eggs

- 1 cup unsweetened coconut milk

- 1/2 teaspoon vanilla extract

- 1 cup mixed berries for filling

- 2 tablespoons unsweetened shredded coconut for garnish

Instructions:

1. In a bowl, whisk together coconut flour, eggs, coconut milk, and vanilla extract until a smooth batter forms.

2. Heat a non-stick skillet over medium heat.

3. Pour 1/4 cup of batter onto the skillet, swirling to spread it thinly.

4. Cook until the edges lift easily, then flip and cook the other side.

5. Repeat with the remaining batter to make multiple crepes.

6. Fill each crepe with mixed berries and fold.

7. Garnish with shredded coconut.

8. Serve warm.

Nutritional Information:

- Calories: 290

- Protein: 11g

- Carbohydrates: 20g

- Fiber: 8g

- Sugars: 6g

- Fat: 18g

- Saturated Fat: 12g

- Sodium: 120mg

8. Turkey and Vegetable Breakfast Skewers

Prep Time: 15 minutes

Cooking Time: 10 minutes

Serving Size: 2

Ingredients:

- 8 ounces turkey breast, cut into cubes

- 1 zucchini, sliced

- 1 red bell pepper, cut into chunks

- 1 tablespoon olive oil

- 1 teaspoon dried oregano

- Salt and pepper to taste

Instructions:

1. Preheat the grill or grill pan over medium-high heat.

2. In a bowl, toss turkey cubes, zucchini slices, and red bell pepper chunks with olive oil, dried oregano, salt, and pepper.

3. Thread the marinated turkey and vegetables onto skewers.

4. Grill the skewers for 5 minutes on each side or until the turkey is cooked through and the vegetables are charred.

5. Serve hot.

Nutritional Information:

- Calories: 320

- Protein: 28g

- Carbohydrates: 10g

- Fiber: 3g

- Sugars: 6g

- Fat: 18g

- Saturated Fat: 3g

- Sodium: 120mg

9. Cauliflower and Broccoli Breakfast Casserole

Prep Time: 20 minutes

Cooking Time: 35 minutes

Serving Size: 4

Ingredients:

- 1 head cauliflower, grated

- 2 cups broccoli florets, chopped

- 6 eggs

- 1/2 cup almond milk

- 1 cup shredded dairy-free cheese

- 1/4 cup nutritional yeast

- 1 teaspoon garlic powder

- Salt and pepper to taste

Instructions:

1. Preheat the oven to 375°F (190°C).

2. In a large bowl, combine grated cauliflower, chopped broccoli, eggs, almond milk, shredded dairy-free cheese, nutritional yeast, garlic powder, salt, and pepper.

3. Transfer the mixture to a greased baking dish.

4. Bake for 35 minutes or until the edges are golden brown and the center is set.

5. Allow the casserole to cool for a few minutes before slicing.

6. Serve warm.

Nutritional Information:

- Calories: 280

- Protein: 15g

- Carbohydrates: 16g

- Fiber: 7g

- Sugars: 5g

- Fat: 18g

- Saturated Fat: 4g

- Sodium: 380mg

10. Pesto and Tomato Breakfast Stuffed Avocado

Prep Time: 10 minutes

Cooking Time: 0 minutes

Serving Size: 2

Ingredients:

- 2 ripe avocados, halved and pitted

- 4 tablespoons lectin-free pesto

- 1 cup cherry tomatoes, halved

- 2 tablespoons pine nuts, toasted

- Fresh basil leaves for garnish

Instructions:

1. Scoop out a small portion of each avocado half to create a hollow for the filling.

2. Spoon 1 tablespoon of lectin-free pesto into each avocado half.

3. Arrange halved cherry tomatoes on top of the pesto.

4. Sprinkle toasted pine nuts over the tomatoes.

5. Garnish with fresh basil leaves.

6. Serve immediately.

Nutritional Information:

- Calories: 320

- Protein: 6g

- Carbohydrates: 16g

- Fiber: 10g

- Sugars: 4g

- Fat: 28g

- Saturated Fat: 4g

- Sodium: 240mg

These lectin-free breakfast recipes provide a variety of delicious and nutritious options to kickstart your day while aligning with your dietary goals. Enjoy exploring these flavorful creations as you prioritize health and wellness in your morning routine.

CHAPTER 4: LUNCH RECIPES

1. Grilled Chicken and Vegetable Salad

Prep Time: 15 minutes

Cooking Time: 15 minutes

Serving Size: 2

Ingredients:

- 2 boneless, skinless chicken breasts

- 4 cups mixed salad greens

- 1 cup cherry tomatoes, halved

- 1 cucumber, sliced

- 1/4 red onion, thinly sliced

- 2 tablespoons olive oil

- 1 tablespoon balsamic vinegar

- Salt and pepper to taste

Instructions:

1. Preheat the grill or grill pan over medium-high heat.

2. Season chicken breasts with salt and pepper.

3. Grill the chicken for 6-8 minutes per side or until fully cooked.

4. In a large bowl, toss salad greens, cherry tomatoes, cucumber, and red onion.

5. Slice grilled chicken and place it on top of the salad.

6. Drizzle with olive oil and balsamic vinegar.

7. Toss the salad to combine all ingredients.

8. Serve immediately.

Nutritional Information:

- Calories: 380

- Protein: 30g

- Carbohydrates: 12g

- Fiber: 4g

- Sugars: 6g

- Fat: 25g

- Saturated Fat: 4g

- Sodium: 160mg

2. Zucchini Noodles with Pesto and Cherry Tomatoes

Prep Time: 20 minutes

Cooking Time: 5 minutes

Serving Size: 2

Ingredients:

- 4 medium zucchinis, spiralized

- 1 cup cherry tomatoes, halved

- 1/4 cup lectin-free pesto

- 2 tablespoons olive oil

- 2 tablespoons pine nuts, toasted

- Fresh basil leaves for garnish

Instructions:

1. Spiralize zucchinis into noodles.

2. In a skillet, heat olive oil over medium heat.

3. Add zucchini noodles and sauté for 3-5 minutes until just tender.

4. Stir in cherry tomatoes and cook for an additional 2 minutes.

5. Toss zucchini noodles and tomatoes with lectin-free pesto.

6. Sprinkle toasted pine nuts over the top.

7. Garnish with fresh basil leaves.

8. Serve warm.

Nutritional Information:

- Calories: 320

- Protein: 8g

- Carbohydrates: 16g

- Fiber: 6g

- Sugars: 8g

- Fat: 25g

- Saturated Fat: 4g

- Sodium: 220mg

3. Salmon and Asparagus Foil Packets

Prep Time: 15 minutes

Cooking Time: 20 minutes

Serving Size: 2

Ingredients:

- 2 salmon fillets

- 1 bunch asparagus, trimmed

- 1 lemon, sliced

- 2 tablespoons olive oil

- 2 cloves garlic, minced

- 1 teaspoon dried dill

- Salt and pepper to taste

Instructions:

1. Preheat the oven to 400°F (200°C).

2. Place each salmon fillet on a piece of foil.

3. Arrange asparagus around the salmon.

4. Drizzle olive oil over the salmon and asparagus.

5. Sprinkle minced garlic and dried dill over the top.

6. Season with salt and pepper.

7. Place lemon slices on top of each salmon fillet.

8. Fold the foil to create sealed packets.

9. Bake for 20 minutes or until the salmon is cooked through.

10. Serve hot.

Nutritional Information:

- Calories: 380

- Protein: 30g

- Carbohydrates: 10g

- Fiber: 4g

- Sugars: 3g

- Fat: 25g

- Saturated Fat: 4g

- Sodium: 160mg

4. Quinoa and Roasted Vegetable Bowl

Prep Time: 15 minutes

Cooking Time: 25 minutes

Serving Size: 2

Ingredients:

- 1 cup quinoa, cooked

- 1 zucchini, diced

- 1 red bell pepper, diced

- 1 cup cherry tomatoes, halved

- 1/4 cup red onion, finely chopped

- 2 tablespoons olive oil

- 1 teaspoon dried oregano

- Salt and pepper to taste

Instructions:

1. Preheat the oven to 400°F (200°C).

2. In a bowl, toss diced zucchini, red bell pepper, cherry tomatoes, and red onion with olive oil and dried oregano.

3. Spread the vegetables on a baking sheet.

4. Roast for 25 minutes or until the vegetables are tender and slightly caramelized.

5. In serving bowls, layer cooked quinoa with the roasted vegetables.

6. Season with salt and pepper.

7. Drizzle with additional olive oil if desired.

8. Serve warm.

Nutritional Information:

- Calories: 420

- Protein: 12g

- Carbohydrates: 65g

- Fiber: 9g

- Sugars: 7g

- Fat: 15g

- Saturated Fat: 2g

- Sodium: 160mg

5. Eggplant and Mushroom Stir-Fry

Prep Time: 20 minutes

Cooking Time: 15 minutes

Serving Size: 2

Ingredients:

- 1 large eggplant, diced

- 2 cups mushrooms, sliced

- 1 red bell pepper, thinly sliced

- 2 tablespoons coconut aminos

- 1 tablespoon olive oil

- 1 teaspoon grated ginger

- 2 cloves garlic, minced

- Sesame seeds for garnish

Instructions:

1. Heat olive oil in a wok or skillet over medium-high heat.

2. Add diced eggplant and stir-fry for 5 minutes until softened.

3. Add sliced mushrooms and red bell pepper to the wok. Continue stir-frying for an additional 5 minutes.

4. In a small bowl, mix coconut aminos, grated ginger, and minced garlic.

5.   Pour the sauce over the vegetables and toss to coat evenly.

6.   Cook for an additional 2-3 minutes until the sauce thickens.

7.   Garnish with sesame seeds.

8.   Serve hot.

Nutritional Information:

- Calories: 300

- Protein: 8g

- Carbohydrates: 25g

- Fiber: 10g

- Sugars: 10g

- Fat: 20g

- Saturated Fat: 3g

- Sodium: 320mg

6. Turkey and Vegetable Lettuce Wraps

Prep Time: 20 minutes

Cooking Time: 10 minutes

Serving Size: 4

Ingredients:

- 1 pound ground turkey

- 1 tablespoon olive oil

- 1 zucchini, diced

- 1 bell pepper, diced

- 1 carrot, julienned

- 4 scallions, sliced

- 2 cloves garlic, minced

- 1/4 cup coconut aminos

- 1 teaspoon sesame oil

- Bibb lettuce leaves for wrapping

Instructions:

1. In a skillet, heat olive oil over medium-high heat.

2. Add ground turkey and cook until browned.

3. Add diced zucchini, bell pepper, carrot, scallions, and minced garlic. Stir-fry for 5 minutes.

4. In a small bowl, mix coconut aminos and sesame oil. Pour over the turkey and vegetables.

5. Cook for an additional 2-3 minutes until the sauce is well incorporated.

6. Spoon the turkey and vegetable mixture onto Bibb lettuce leaves.

7. Serve immediately.

Nutritional Information:

- Calories: 320

- Protein: 25g

- Carbohydrates: 12g

- Fiber: 4g

- Sugars: 6g

- Fat: 20g

- Saturated Fat: 4g

- Sodium: 260mg

7. Cabbage and Chicken Stir-Fry

Prep Time: 15 minutes

Cooking Time: 15 minutes

Serving Size: 2

Ingredients:

- 2 boneless, skinless chicken breasts, thinly sliced

- 1 small cabbage, shredded

- 1 cup snap peas, trimmed

- 1 carrot, julienned

- 2 tablespoons coconut aminos

- 1 tablespoon olive oil

- 1 teaspoon grated ginger

- 2 cloves garlic, minced

Instructions:

1. In a wok or large skillet, heat olive oil over medium-high heat.

2. Add sliced chicken and stir-fry until cooked through.

3. Add shredded cabbage, snap peas, and julienned carrot to the wok. Continue stir-frying for 5 minutes.

4. In a small bowl, mix coconut aminos, grated ginger, and minced garlic.

5. Pour the sauce over the chicken and vegetables. Toss to coat evenly.

6. Cook for an additional 2-3 minutes until the sauce thickens.

7. Serve hot.

Nutritional Information:

- Calories: 350

- Protein: 30g

- Carbohydrates: 18g

- Fiber: 8g

- Sugars: 10g

- Fat: 18g

- Saturated Fat: 3g

- Sodium: 380mg

8. Cauliflower Rice and Shrimp Bowl

Prep Time: 20 minutes

Cooking Time: 10 minutes

Serving Size: 2

Ingredients:

- 1 pound shrimp, peeled and deveined

- 4 cups cauliflower rice, cooked

- 1 cup broccoli florets, steamed

- 1 bell pepper, diced

- 2 tablespoons coconut oil

- 2 tablespoons coconut aminos

- 1 teaspoon sesame oil

- 1 teaspoon minced garlic

Instructions:

1. In a large skillet, heat coconut oil over medium-high heat.

2. Add shrimp and cook until pink and opaque.

3. Add diced bell pepper and steamed broccoli to the skillet. Stir-fry for 3 minutes.

4. In a small bowl, mix coconut aminos, sesame oil, and minced garlic.

5. Pour the sauce over the shrimp and vegetables. Toss to combine.

6. In serving bowls, layer cauliflower rice with the shrimp and vegetable mixture.

7. Serve warm.

Nutritional Information:

- Calories: 380

- Protein: 30g

- Carbohydrates: 20g

- Fiber: 8g

- Sugars: 6g

- Fat: 20g

- Saturated Fat: 12g

- Sodium: 420mg

9. Lentil and Vegetable Soup

Prep Time: 15 minutes

Cooking Time: 30 minutes

Serving Size: 4

Ingredients:

- 1 cup green lentils, rinsed

- 1 onion, diced

- 2 carrots, sliced

- 2 celery stalks, chopped

- 3 cloves garlic, minced

- 6 cups vegetable broth

- 1 teaspoon ground cumin

- 1 teaspoon smoked paprika

- Salt and pepper to taste

- Fresh parsley for garnish

Instructions:

1. In a large pot, sauté diced onion, sliced carrots, chopped celery, and minced garlic until softened.

2. Add rinsed green lentils to the pot.

3. Pour in vegetable broth and season with ground cumin, smoked paprika, salt, and pepper.

4. Bring the soup to a boil, then reduce heat and simmer for 25-30 minutes until lentils are tender.

5. Garnish with fresh parsley before serving.

6. Serve hot.

Nutritional Information:

- Calories: 280

- Protein: 18g

- Carbohydrates: 45g

- Fiber: 16g

- Sugars: 5g

- Fat: 2g

- Saturated Fat: 0g

- Sodium: 920mg

10. Butternut Squash and Chicken Stew

Prep Time: 20 minutes

Cooking Time: 35 minutes

Serving Size: 4

Ingredients:

- 1 pound chicken thighs, boneless and skinless, diced

- 4 cups butternut squash, peeled and cubed

- 1 onion, diced

- 3 cloves garlic, minced

- 4 cups chicken broth

- 1 teaspoon dried thyme

- 1 teaspoon ground turmeric

- Salt and pepper to taste

- Fresh sage for garnish

Instructions:

1. In a large pot, sauté diced chicken until browned.

2. Add diced onion and minced garlic. Cook until softened.

3. Stir in cubed butternut squash.

4. Pour in chicken broth and season with dried thyme, ground turmeric, salt, and pepper.

5. Bring the stew to a boil, then reduce heat and simmer for 30-35 minutes until the butternut squash is tender.

6. Garnish with fresh sage before serving.

7. Serve hot.

Nutritional Information:

- Calories: 320

- Protein: 22g

- Carbohydrates: 30g

- Fiber: 8g

- Sugars: 5g

- Fat: 15g

- Saturated Fat: 4g

- Sodium: 820mg

These lectin-free lunch recipes offer a delightful range of flavors and nutritional benefits, ensuring that you enjoy a satisfying and health-conscious midday meal. Feel free to explore these options to enhance your lectin-free journey.

CHAPTER 5: DINNER RECIPES

1. Baked Lemon Herb Chicken

Prep Time: 15 minutes

Cooking Time: 30 minutes

Serving Size: 4

Ingredients:

- 4 boneless, skinless chicken breasts

- 2 lemons, juiced and zested

- 3 tablespoons olive oil

- 2 cloves garlic, minced

- 1 teaspoon dried thyme

- 1 teaspoon dried rosemary

- Salt and pepper to taste

- Fresh parsley for garnish

Instructions:

1. Preheat the oven to 400°F (200°C).

2. In a bowl, mix lemon juice, lemon zest, olive oil, minced garlic, dried thyme, dried rosemary, salt, and pepper.

3. Place chicken breasts in a baking dish and pour the lemon herb mixture over them.

4. Bake for 25-30 minutes or until the chicken is cooked through.

5. Garnish with fresh parsley before serving.

6. Serve hot.

Nutritional Information:

- Calories: 280

- Protein: 30g

- Carbohydrates: 2g

- Fiber: 1g

- Sugars: 0g

- Fat: 16g

- Saturated Fat: 3g

- Sodium: 120mg

2. Cauliflower Alfredo with Shrimp and Spinach

Prep Time: 20 minutes

Cooking Time: 15 minutes

Serving Size: 4

Ingredients:

- 1 pound shrimp, peeled and deveined

- 1 large cauliflower, cut into florets

- 2 cups spinach, chopped

- 2 cloves garlic, minced

- 1 cup almond milk

- 1/4 cup nutritional yeast

- 2 tablespoons olive oil

- Salt and pepper to taste

- Fresh basil for garnish

Instructions:

1. Cook cauliflower florets until tender, then blend with almond milk, nutritional yeast, salt, and pepper to create a creamy sauce.

2. In a skillet, heat olive oil over medium-high heat.

3. Add minced garlic and shrimp, cooking until the shrimp are pink and opaque.

4. Stir in chopped spinach until wilted.

5. Pour the cauliflower Alfredo sauce over the shrimp and spinach, stirring to combine.

6. Cook for an additional 2-3 minutes until heated through.

7. Garnish with fresh basil.

8. Serve warm.

Nutritional Information:

- Calories: 320

- Protein: 28g

- Carbohydrates: 10g

- Fiber: 5g

- Sugars: 2g

- Fat: 18g

- Saturated Fat: 3g

- Sodium: 320mg

3. Turkey and Vegetable Stuffed Bell Peppers

Prep Time: 20 minutes

Cooking Time: 40 minutes

Serving Size: 4

Ingredients:

- 1 pound ground turkey

- 4 bell peppers, halved and seeds removed

- 1 cup cauliflower rice

- 1 zucchini, diced

- 1 cup tomato sauce

- 1 teaspoon dried oregano

- 1 teaspoon garlic powder

- Salt and pepper to taste

- Fresh parsley for garnish

Instructions:

1. Preheat the oven to 375°F (190°C).

2. In a skillet, cook ground turkey until browned.

3. Add cauliflower rice, diced zucchini, tomato sauce, dried oregano, garlic powder, salt, and pepper. Mix well.

4. Stuff each bell pepper half with the turkey and vegetable mixture.

5. Place the stuffed peppers in a baking dish.

6. Bake for 30-35 minutes or until the peppers are tender.

7. Garnish with fresh parsley before serving.

8. Serve hot.

Nutritional Information:

- Calories: 290

- Protein: 25g

- Carbohydrates: 15g

- Fiber: 5g

- Sugars: 8g

- Fat: 15g

- Saturated Fat: 3g

- Sodium: 340mg

4. Baked Salmon with Dill and Lemon

Prep Time: 10 minutes

Cooking Time: 20 minutes

Serving Size: 2

Ingredients:

- 2 salmon fillets

- 2 tablespoons olive oil

- 1 lemon, sliced

- 2 tablespoons fresh dill, chopped

- Salt and pepper to taste

Instructions:

1. Preheat the oven to 400°F (200°C).

2. Place salmon fillets on a baking sheet.

3. Drizzle olive oil over the salmon and season with salt and pepper.

4. Place lemon slices on top of each salmon fillet.

5. Sprinkle fresh dill over the top.

6. Bake for 15-20 minutes or until the salmon is cooked through.

7. Serve hot.

Nutritional Information:

- Calories: 320

- Protein: 30g

- Carbohydrates: 2g

- Fiber: 1g

- Sugars: 0g

- Fat: 22g

- Saturated Fat: 4g

- Sodium: 160mg

5. Eggplant Lasagna

Prep Time: 30 minutes

Cooking Time: 45 minutes

Serving Size: 6

Ingredients:

- 1 large eggplant, sliced lengthwise

- 1 pound ground beef

- 2 cups tomato sauce

- 1 cup dairy-free ricotta cheese

- 1 cup baby spinach

- 1 teaspoon dried basil

- 1 teaspoon dried oregano

- Salt and pepper to taste

- 1 cup dairy-free mozzarella, shredded

Instructions:

1. Preheat the oven to 375°F (190°C).

2. Grill or roast eggplant slices until softened.

3. In a skillet, cook ground beef until browned.

4. Mix ground beef with tomato sauce, dried basil, dried oregano, salt, and pepper.

5. In a baking dish, layer eggplant slices, beef and tomato sauce mixture, dairy-free ricotta, and baby spinach.

6. Repeat the layers, finishing with a layer of eggplant on top.

7. Sprinkle dairy-free mozzarella on top.

8. Bake for 30-35 minutes or until bubbly and golden.

9. Let it cool for a few minutes before serving.

10. Serve warm.

Nutritional Information:

- Calories: 380

- Protein: 28g

- Carbohydrates: 15g

- Fiber: 6g

- Sugars: 8g

- Fat: 22g

- Saturated Fat: 6g

- Sodium: 540mg

6. Spaghetti Squash with Turkey Bolognese

Prep Time: 20 minutes

Cooking Time: 50 minutes

Serving Size: 4

Ingredients:

- 1 large spaghetti squash, halved and seeds removed

- 1 pound ground turkey

- 1 onion, diced

- 2 cloves garlic, minced

- 1 cup tomato sauce

- 1 teaspoon dried oregano

- 1 teaspoon dried basil

- Salt and pepper to taste

- Fresh basil for garnish

Instructions:

1. Preheat the oven to 375°F (190°C).

2. Roast spaghetti squash halves, cut side down, for 40-45 minutes or until tender.

3. In a skillet, cook ground turkey until browned.

4. Add diced onion and minced garlic, cooking until softened.

5. Stir in tomato sauce, dried oregano, dried basil, salt, and pepper.

6. Use a fork to scrape the cooked spaghetti squash into "noodles."

7. Serve the turkey Bolognese over the spaghetti squash.

8. Garnish with fresh basil.

9. Serve hot.

Nutritional Information:

- Calories: 320

- Protein: 25g

- Carbohydrates: 15g

- Fiber: 4g

- Sugars: 6g

- Fat: 18g

- Saturated Fat: 3g

- Sodium: 340mg

7. Lemon Garlic Shrimp and Broccoli Stir-Fry

Prep Time: 15 minutes

Cooking Time: 10 minutes

Serving Size: 2

Ingredients:

- 1 pound shrimp, peeled and deveined

- 2 cups broccoli florets

- 2 tablespoons olive oil

- 3 cloves garlic, minced

- 1 lemon, juiced and zested

- Salt and pepper to taste

- Red pepper flakes for spice (optional)

Instructions:

1. In a wok or large skillet, heat olive oil over medium-high heat.

2. Add minced garlic and sauté until fragrant.

3. Add shrimp and cook until pink and opaque.

4. Stir in broccoli florets and cook for an additional 3-5 minutes until tender-crisp.

5. Pour lemon juice and zest over the shrimp and broccoli.

6. Season with salt, pepper, and red pepper flakes if desired.

7. Toss to coat evenly.

8. Serve hot.

Nutritional Information:

- Calories: 280

- Protein: 30g

- Carbohydrates: 10g

- Fiber: 3g

- Sugars: 3g

- Fat: 14g

- Saturated Fat: 2g

- Sodium: 260mg

8. Stuffed Acorn Squash with Ground Bison

Prep Time: 25 minutes

Cooking Time: 45 minutes

Serving Size: 4

Ingredients:

- 2 acorn squash, halved and seeds removed

- 1 pound ground bison

- 1 cup cauliflower rice

- 1/2 cup diced tomatoes

- 1/4 cup chopped red onion

- 1 teaspoon ground cumin

- 1 teaspoon chili powder

- Salt and pepper to taste

- Fresh cilantro for garnish

Instructions:

1. Preheat the oven to 375°F (190°C).

2. Roast acorn squash halves, cut side down, for 30-35 minutes or until tender.

3. In a skillet, cook ground bison until browned.

4. Add cauliflower rice, diced tomatoes, chopped red onion, ground cumin, chili powder, salt, and pepper. Mix well.

5. Stuff each acorn squash half with the bison and vegetable mixture.

6. Bake for an additional 15 minutes.

7. Garnish with fresh cilantro before serving.

8. Serve hot.

Nutritional Information:

- Calories: 320

- Protein: 28g

- Carbohydrates: 20g

- Fiber: 6g

- Sugars: 4g

- Fat: 16g

- Saturated Fat: 5g

- Sodium: 380mg

9. Garlic Herb Roasted Chicken Thighs

Prep Time: 10 minutes

Cooking Time: 40 minutes

Serving Size: 4

Ingredients:

- 8 chicken thighs, bone-in and skin-on

- 3 tablespoons olive oil

- 4 cloves garlic, minced

- 1 teaspoon dried thyme

- 1 teaspoon dried rosemary

- 1 teaspoon dried sage

- Salt and pepper to taste

- Fresh parsley for garnish

Instructions:

1. Preheat the oven to 400°F (200°C).

2. In a bowl, mix olive oil, minced garlic, dried thyme, dried rosemary, dried sage, salt, and pepper.

3. Rub the chicken thighs with the herb mixture, ensuring they are well coated.

4. Place the chicken thighs on a baking sheet.

5. Roast for 35-40 minutes or until the chicken is golden brown and cooked through.

6. Garnish with fresh parsley before serving.

7. Serve hot.

Nutritional Information:

- Calories: 380

- Protein: 30g

- Carbohydrates: 0g

- Fiber: 0g

- Sugars: 0g

- Fat: 28g

- Saturated Fat: 6g

- Sodium: 180mg

10. Mushroom and Spinach Stuffed Chicken Breasts

Prep Time: 25 minutes

Cooking Time: 30 minutes

Serving Size: 4

Ingredients:

- 4 boneless, skinless chicken breasts

- 2 cups mushrooms, finely chopped

- 2 cups spinach, chopped

- 1/2 cup almond flour

- 2 tablespoons olive oil

- 2 cloves garlic, minced

- 1 teaspoon dried thyme

- Salt and pepper to taste

- Lemon wedges for serving

Instructions:

1. Preheat the oven to 375°F (190°C).

2. In a skillet, heat olive oil over medium-high heat.

3. Add minced garlic and sauté until fragrant.

4. Add chopped mushrooms and cook until they release their moisture.

5. Stir in chopped spinach, almond flour, dried thyme, salt, and pepper. Cook until the mixture is well combined and slightly thickened.

6. Make a pocket in each chicken breast and stuff with the mushroom and spinach mixture.

7. Place the stuffed chicken breasts in a baking dish.

8. Bake for 25-30 minutes or until the chicken is cooked through.

9. Serve with lemon wedges on the side.

10. Serve hot.

Nutritional Information:

- Calories: 320

- Protein: 30g

- Carbohydrates: 6g

- Fiber: 2g

- Sugars: 2g

- Fat: 20g

- Saturated Fat: 4g

- Sodium: 220mg

These lectin-free dinner recipes are not only delicious but also nutritionally balanced, providing a satisfying and wholesome conclusion to your day. Enjoy exploring these flavorful options as you prioritize health and wellness in your meals.

CHAPTER 6: SNACK AND DESSERT RECIPES

1. Almond Butter Energy Bites

Prep Time: 15 minutes

Cooking Time: 0 minutes

Serving Size: 12 bites

Ingredients:

- 1 cup almond butter

- 1/2 cup coconut flour

- 1/4 cup honey or maple syrup

- 1 teaspoon vanilla extract

- Pinch of sea salt

- Optional: shredded coconut for coating

Instructions:

1. In a mixing bowl, combine almond butter, coconut flour, honey or maple syrup, vanilla extract, and a pinch of sea salt.

2. Mix until well combined.

3. Roll the mixture into small, bite-sized balls.

4. Optional: Roll the energy bites in shredded coconut for added texture.

5. Refrigerate for at least 30 minutes before serving.

6. Serve chilled.

Nutritional Information:

- Calories: 120 per energy bite

- Protein: 4g

- Carbohydrates: 8g

- Fiber: 2g

- Sugars: 4g

- Fat: 9g

- Saturated Fat: 1g

- Sodium: 30mg

2. Chocolate Avocado Mousse

Prep Time: 10 minutes

Cooking Time: 0 minutes

Serving Size: 4

Ingredients:

- 2 ripe avocados

- 1/4 cup cocoa powder

- 1/4 cup honey or maple syrup

- 1 teaspoon vanilla extract

- Pinch of sea salt

- Berries for garnish

Instructions:

1. In a blender or food processor, combine ripe avocados, cocoa powder, honey or maple syrup, vanilla extract, and a pinch of sea salt.

2. Blend until smooth and creamy.

3. Refrigerate for at least 1 hour before serving.

4. Garnish with fresh berries.

5. Serve chilled.

Nutritional Information:

- Calories: 220 per serving

- Protein: 3g

- Carbohydrates: 20g

- Fiber: 8g

- Sugars: 10g

- Fat: 15g

- Saturated Fat: 2g

- Sodium: 10mg

3. Cinnamon Almond Roasted Chickpeas

Prep Time: 10 minutes

Cooking Time: 30 minutes

Serving Size: 4

Ingredients:

- 2 cups cooked chickpeas, dried and patted dry

- 2 tablespoons almond oil

- 1 teaspoon ground cinnamon

- 1/4 teaspoon sea salt

- 1 tablespoon honey or maple syrup (optional)

Instructions:

1. Preheat the oven to 400°F (200°C).

2. In a bowl, toss dried chickpeas with almond oil, ground cinnamon, and sea salt.

3. Spread the chickpeas on a baking sheet in a single layer.

4. Roast for 30 minutes or until crispy, shaking the pan halfway through.

5. Optional: Drizzle honey or maple syrup over the chickpeas and toss to coat.

6. Allow to cool before serving.

7. Serve at room temperature.

Nutritional Information:

- Calories: 180 per serving

- Protein: 6g

- Carbohydrates: 24g

- Fiber: 6g

- Sugars: 3g

- Fat: 8g

- Saturated Fat: 1g

- Sodium: 150mg

4. Berry Chia Seed Pudding

Prep Time: 10 minutes (plus overnight chilling)

Cooking Time: 0 minutes

Serving Size: 2

Ingredients:

- 1/2 cup chia seeds

- 2 cups almond milk

- 1 tablespoon honey or maple syrup

- 1 teaspoon vanilla extract

- 1 cup mixed berries

Instructions:

1. In a bowl, mix chia seeds, almond milk, honey or maple syrup, and vanilla extract.

2. Stir well and refrigerate overnight or for at least 4 hours.

3. Before serving, stir the chia pudding to ensure it's well-set.

4. Spoon the pudding into serving bowls and top with mixed berries.

5. Serve chilled.

Nutritional Information:

- Calories: 180 per serving

- Protein: 5g

- Carbohydrates: 25g

- Fiber: 12g

- Sugars: 10g

- Fat: 7g

- Saturated Fat: 1g

- Sodium: 100mg

5. Coconut Flour Banana Bread

Prep Time: 15 minutes

Cooking Time: 40 minutes

Serving Size: 8 slices

Ingredients:

- 3 ripe bananas, mashed

- 4 eggs

- 1/4 cup coconut oil, melted

- 1 teaspoon vanilla extract

- 1/2 cup coconut flour

- 1 teaspoon baking soda

- Pinch of sea salt

- 1/2 cup chopped walnuts (optional)

Instructions:

1. Preheat the oven to 350°F (180°C). Grease a loaf pan.

2. In a bowl, mix mashed bananas, eggs, melted coconut oil, and vanilla extract.

3. In a separate bowl, combine coconut flour, baking soda, and a pinch of sea salt.

4. Gradually add the dry ingredients to the wet ingredients, stirring until well combined.

5. Fold in chopped walnuts if using.

6. Pour the batter into the prepared loaf pan.

7. Bake for 35-40 minutes or until a toothpick inserted comes out clean.

8. Allow to cool before slicing.

9. Serve at room temperature.

Nutritional Information:

- Calories: 160 per slice

- Protein: 4g

- Carbohydrates: 15g

- Fiber: 4g

- Sugars: 7g

- Fat: 10g

- Saturated Fat: 7g

- Sodium: 180mg

6. Vanilla Almond Date Balls

Prep Time: 20 minutes

Cooking Time: 0 minutes

Serving Size: 12 balls

Ingredients:

- 1 cup almonds

- 1 cup pitted dates

- 1 teaspoon vanilla extract

- Pinch of sea salt

- Shredded coconut for coating

Instructions:

1. In a food processor, blend almonds until finely ground.

2. Add pitted dates, vanilla extract, and a pinch of sea salt. Blend until a sticky dough forms.

3. Roll the mixture into small balls.

4. Roll the date balls in shredded coconut to coat.

5. Refrigerate for at least 30 minutes before serving.

6. Serve chilled.

Nutritional Information:

- Calories: 90 per ball

- Protein: 2g

- Carbohydrates: 10g

- Fiber: 2g

- Sugars: 7g

- Fat: 5g

- Saturated Fat: 0g

- Sodium: 0mg

7. Apple Cinnamon Walnut Muffins

Prep Time: 15 minutes

Cooking Time: 25 minutes

Serving Size: 6 muffins

Ingredients:

- 2 cups almond flour

- 1 teaspoon baking soda

- 1/2 teaspoon ground cinnamon

- Pinch of sea salt

- 3 eggs

- 1/4 cup coconut oil, melted

- 1/4 cup honey or maple syrup

- 1 teaspoon vanilla extract

- 1 apple, peeled and diced

- 1/2 cup chopped walnuts

Instructions:

1. Preheat the oven to 350°F (180°C). Line a muffin tin with paper liners.

2. In a bowl, whisk together almond flour, baking soda, ground cinnamon, and a pinch of sea salt.

3. In a separate bowl, beat eggs and add melted coconut oil, honey or maple syrup, and vanilla extract.

4. Gradually add the wet ingredients to the dry ingredients, stirring until just combined.

5. Fold in diced apple and chopped walnuts.

6. Spoon the batter into the muffin tin.

7. Bake for 20-25 minutes or until a toothpick inserted comes out clean.

8. Allow to cool before serving.

9. Serve at room temperature.

Nutritional Information:

- Calories: 280 per muffin

- Protein: 8g

- Carbohydrates: 18g

- Fiber: 4g

- Sugars: 11g

- Fat: 20g

- Saturated Fat: 5g

- Sodium: 180mg

8. Pecan Pie Energy Bars

Prep Time: 20 minutes

Cooking Time: 0 minutes

Serving Size: 8 bars

Ingredients:

- 1 cup pecans

- 1 cup dates, pitted

- 1/4 cup almond butter

- 1 teaspoon vanilla extract

- Pinch of sea salt

Instructions:

1. In a food processor, blend pecans until finely ground.

2. Add pitted dates, almond butter, vanilla extract, and a pinch of sea salt. Blend until a sticky dough forms.

3. Press the mixture into a lined baking dish to form an even layer.

4. Refrigerate for at least 1 hour before cutting into bars.

5. Serve chilled.

Nutritional Information:

- Calories: 180 per bar

- Protein: 3g

- Carbohydrates: 18g

- Fiber: 4g

- Sugars: 12g

- Fat: 12g

- Saturated Fat: 1g

- Sodium: 20mg

9. Lemon Poppy Seed Coconut Flour Cookies

Prep Time: 15 minutes

Cooking Time: 10 minutes

Serving Size: 12 cookies

Ingredients:

- 1/2 cup coconut flour

- 1/4 cup coconut oil, melted

- 1/4 cup honey or maple syrup

- 2 eggs

- 1 lemon, juiced and zested

- 1 teaspoon vanilla extract

- 1 tablespoon poppy seeds

- Pinch of sea salt

Instructions:

1. Preheat the oven to 350°F (180°C). Line a baking sheet with parchment paper.

2. In a bowl, mix coconut flour, melted coconut oil, honey or maple syrup, eggs, lemon juice, lemon zest, vanilla extract, poppy seeds, and a pinch of sea salt.

3. Drop spoonfuls of the batter onto the prepared baking sheet.

4. Bake for 8-10 minutes or until the edges are golden brown.

5. Allow to cool before serving.

6. Serve at room temperature.

Nutritional Information:

- Calories: 80 per cookie

- Protein: 2g

- Carbohydrates: 8g

- Fiber: 2g

- Sugars: 5g

- Fat: 5g

- Saturated Fat: 4g

- Sodium: 30mg

10. Pumpkin Spice Pecan Cookies

Prep Time: 20 minutes

Cooking Time: 12 minutes

Serving Size: 10 cookies

Ingredients:

- 1 cup almond flour

- 1/4 cup coconut oil, melted

- 1/4 cup pumpkin puree

- 1/4 cup coconut sugar

- 1 teaspoon pumpkin spice

- 1/2 cup chopped pecans

- Pinch of sea salt

Instructions:

1. Preheat the oven to 350°F (180°C). Line a baking sheet with parchment paper.

2. In a bowl, mix almond flour, melted coconut oil, pumpkin puree, coconut sugar, pumpkin spice, chopped pecans, and a pinch of sea salt.

3. Drop spoonfuls of the batter onto the prepared baking sheet.

4. Flatten each cookie slightly with the back of a spoon.

5. Bake for 10-12 minutes or until the edges are golden brown.

6. Allow to cool before serving.

7. Serve at room temperature.

Nutritional Information:

- Calories: 120 per cookie

- Protein: 3g

- Carbohydrates: 7g

- Fiber: 2g

- Sugars: 4g

- Fat: 10g

- Saturated Fat: 3g

- Sodium: 40mg

These delightful lectin-free snack and dessert recipes offer a range of flavors and textures, ensuring you can enjoy a sweet treat without compromising your dietary preferences. Feel free to indulge in these wholesome options for a satisfying snack or a guilt-free dessert.

CHAPTER 7: MEAL PLANNING AND PREPPING

Weekly Meal Plans

Meal planning is a cornerstone of successful adherence to a lectin-free diet. Crafting thoughtful weekly meal plans not only saves time but also ensures that your nutritional needs are met. It's an opportunity to introduce variety into your diet while maintaining the principles of lectin avoidance.

Importance of Weekly Meal Plans

Creating a weekly meal plan provides structure and organization to your dietary habits. It helps in achieving nutritional balance by incorporating a diverse range of lectin-free foods. With a well-thought-out plan, you can ensure that each meal offers a mix of proteins, healthy fats, and nutrient-rich vegetables.

How to Create a Lectin-Free Weekly Meal Plan

1. **Assess Dietary Preferences and Restrictions:** Consider your taste preferences, dietary restrictions, and any specific health goals you might have. This initial assessment sets the stage for a personalized and sustainable meal plan.

2. **Include a Variety of Vegetables:** Diversify your vegetable intake to maximize nutrient intake. Include leafy greens,

cruciferous vegetables, colorful bell peppers, and other lectin-free options. Rotate these throughout the week to provide a spectrum of vitamins and minerals.

3. **Incorporate Lean Proteins:** Opt for lean protein sources such as poultry, fish, and plant-based proteins like lentils and legumes that have been properly prepared. Variety in protein sources ensures a broad range of amino acids and nutrients.

4. **Integrate Healthy Fats:** Include sources of healthy fats like avocados, olive oil, and nuts. These not only contribute to the overall flavor of your meals but also provide essential fatty acids crucial for overall health.

5. **Plan Balanced Meals:** Aim for balanced meals that combine proteins, fats, and carbohydrates. This balance helps in stabilizing blood sugar levels and sustaining energy throughout the day.

6. **Consider Portion Sizes:** Be mindful of portion sizes to avoid overeating. Adjust portion sizes based on individual factors such as age, activity level, and specific health goals.

7. **Plan for Snacks:** Incorporate healthy snacks between meals to prevent unnecessary hunger and potential cravings for non-compliant foods. Snacks can include fresh fruit, raw vegetables with hummus, or a handful of nuts.

8. **Prepare a Shopping List:** Once your meal plan is finalized, create a comprehensive shopping list. This reduces the

likelihood of impulse purchases and ensures you have all the necessary ingredients on hand.

9. **Prep Ingredients in Advance:** If time allows, consider prepping some ingredients in advance. Chop vegetables, marinate proteins, or prepare lectin-free sauces and dressings to streamline the cooking process during the week.

10. **Flexibility for Special Occasions:** While planning is essential, allow room for flexibility. If unexpected events or invitations arise, having a plan for quick and compliant meals ensures you stay on track even during busy days.

Batch Cooking for Efficiency

Batch cooking is a valuable strategy for optimizing your time and effort in the kitchen. It involves preparing larger quantities of food at once and storing portions for future meals. This approach is particularly beneficial for those following a lectin-free diet, as it minimizes daily cooking while still providing access to wholesome, home-cooked meals.

Advantages of Batch Cooking

1. **Time Efficiency:** Batch cooking saves time in the long run by consolidating meal preparation. Spending a few hours on a weekend or designated day to cook in larger quantities reduces the time spent cooking on busy weekdays.

2. **Consistent Meal Quality:** Cooking in batches allows for consistent portion control and flavor. You can ensure that each

serving contains the right balance of lectin-free ingredients, maintaining the integrity of your dietary choices.

3. **Minimizes Food Waste:** By preparing larger quantities, you can buy ingredients in bulk, reducing packaging and minimizing food waste. Additionally, leftovers can be frozen for future use, preventing unused ingredients from going bad.

4. **Budget-Friendly:** Batch cooking often proves to be cost-effective. Buying ingredients in bulk tends to be less expensive, and cooking at home saves money compared to dining out regularly.

5. **Convenient Meal Options:** Having pre-cooked portions in the refrigerator or freezer provides convenient options for meals when you're short on time. This reduces the temptation to opt for less healthy, convenience foods.

How to Incorporate Batch Cooking into Your Routine

1. **Choose Batch-Friendly Recipes:** Select recipes that lend themselves well to batch cooking. Dishes like stews, casseroles, and soups are excellent candidates as they often improve in flavor over time.

2. **Invest in Storage Containers:** Ensure you have a variety of airtight containers suitable for freezing. Glass containers are an excellent choice for both reheating and preserving the quality of your batch-cooked meals.

3. **Label and Date:** Properly label each container with the contents and date of preparation. This helps you keep track of freshness and ensures you rotate older items first.

4. **Plan a Batch Cooking Day:** Dedicate a specific day or time during the week for batch cooking. This can be a weekend afternoon or a less hectic weekday evening. Having a designated time ensures consistency.

5. **Rotate Menu Items:** While batch cooking provides convenience, it's essential to maintain variety in your diet. Rotate through different recipes each week to prevent monotony and ensure you receive a broad spectrum of nutrients.

6. **Include Freezer-Friendly Ingredients:** Choose ingredients that freeze well. Some vegetables, grains, and proteins may have different textures when thawed, so it's crucial to experiment and discover what works best for your preferences.

7. **Mindful Thawing:** Plan ahead for thawing frozen meals. Transfer items from the freezer to the refrigerator the night before to allow for gradual thawing, preserving the quality of the food.

8. **Explore One-Pot Meals:** Simplify your batch cooking by exploring one-pot meals. These often require less cleanup and can be easily scaled up to provide multiple servings.

CHAPTER 8: 28-DAY MEAL PLAN

This concludes the 28-day lectin-free meal plan, ensuring each day brings a unique combination of flavors and nutrients. Feel free to swap out meals, adjust portions, or introduce new recipes based on personal preferences and nutritional needs. Remember to stay mindful of hydration and listen to your body's signals for hunger and satisfaction. Enjoy your journey to a healthier lifestyle with this diverse and delicious lectin-free meal plan!

Day 1:

- **Breakfast:** Lectin-Free Berry Smoothie Bowl

- **Lunch:** Grilled Chicken and Vegetable Salad

- **Dinner:** Baked Lemon Herb Chicken

- **Snack/Dessert:** Almond Butter Energy Bites

Day 2:

- **Breakfast:** Spinach and Tomato Omelette

- **Lunch:** Zucchini Noodles with Pesto and Cherry Tomatoes

- **Dinner:** Cauliflower Alfredo with Shrimp and Spinach

- **Snack/Dessert:** Chocolate Avocado Mousse

Day 3:

- **Breakfast:** Almond Flour Pancakes

- **Lunch:** Salmon and Asparagus Foil Packets

- **Dinner:** Turkey and Vegetable Stuffed Bell Peppers

- **Snack/Dessert:** Cinnamon Almond Roasted Chickpeas

Day 4:

- **Breakfast:** Avocado and Smoked Salmon Breakfast Wrap

- **Lunch:** Quinoa and Roasted Vegetable Bowl

- **Dinner:** Baked Salmon with Dill and Lemon

- **Snack/Dessert:** Berry Chia Seed Pudding

Day 5:

- **Breakfast:** Chia Seed Pudding Parfait

- **Lunch:** Eggplant and Mushroom Stir-Fry

- **Dinner:** Eggplant Lasagna

- **Snack/Dessert:** Coconut Flour Banana Bread

Day 6:

- **Breakfast:** Sweet Potato and Kale Breakfast Hash

- **Lunch:** Turkey and Vegetable Lettuce Wraps

- **Dinner:** Spaghetti Squash with Turkey Bolognese

- **Snack/Dessert:** Vanilla Almond Date Balls

Day 7:

- **Breakfast:** Coconut Flour Crepes with Berries

- **Lunch:** Cabbage and Chicken Stir-Fry

- **Dinner:** Lemon Garlic Shrimp and Broccoli Stir-Fry

- **Snack/Dessert:** Apple Cinnamon Walnut Muffins

Day 8:

- **Breakfast:** Turkey and Vegetable Breakfast Skewers

- **Lunch:** Cauliflower Rice and Shrimp Bowl

- **Dinner:** Stuffed Acorn Squash with Ground Bison

- **Snack/Dessert:** Pecan Pie Energy Bars

Day 9:

- **Breakfast:** Cauliflower and Broccoli Breakfast Casserole

- **Lunch:** Lentil and Vegetable Soup

- **Dinner:** Garlic Herb Roasted Chicken Thighs

- **Snack/Dessert:** Lemon Poppy Seed Coconut Flour Cookies

Day 10:

- **Breakfast:** Pesto and Tomato Breakfast Stuffed Avocado

- **Lunch:** Butternut Squash and Chicken Stew

- **Dinner:** Mushroom and Spinach Stuffed Chicken Breasts

- **Snack/Dessert:** Pumpkin Spice Pecan Cookies

Day 11:

- **Breakfast:** Lectin-Free Berry Smoothie Bowl

- **Lunch:** Grilled Chicken and Vegetable Salad

- **Dinner:** Baked Lemon Herb Chicken

- **Snack/Dessert:** Almond Butter Energy Bites

Day 12:

- **Breakfast:** Spinach and Tomato Omelette

- **Lunch:** Zucchini Noodles with Pesto and Cherry Tomatoes

- **Dinner:** Cauliflower Alfredo with Shrimp and Spinach

- **Snack/Dessert:** Chocolate Avocado Mousse

Day 13:

- **Breakfast:** Almond Flour Pancakes

- **Lunch:** Salmon and Asparagus Foil Packets

- **Dinner:** Turkey and Vegetable Stuffed Bell Peppers

- **Snack/Dessert:** Cinnamon Almond Roasted Chickpeas

Day 14:

- **Breakfast:** Avocado and Smoked Salmon Breakfast Wrap

- **Lunch:** Quinoa and Roasted Vegetable Bowl

- **Dinner:** Baked Salmon with Dill and Lemon

- **Snack/Dessert:** Berry Chia Seed Pudding

Day 15:

- **Breakfast:** Chia Seed Pudding Parfait

- **Lunch:** Eggplant and Mushroom Stir-Fry

- **Dinner:** Eggplant Lasagna

- **Snack/Dessert:** Coconut Flour Banana Bread

Day 16:

- **Breakfast:** Sweet Potato and Kale Breakfast Hash

- **Lunch:** Turkey and Vegetable Lettuce Wraps

- **Dinner:** Spaghetti Squash with Turkey Bolognese

- **Snack/Dessert:** Vanilla Almond Date Balls

Day 17:

- **Breakfast:** Coconut Flour Crepes with Berries

- **Lunch:** Cabbage and Chicken Stir-Fry

- **Dinner:** Lemon Garlic Shrimp and Broccoli Stir-Fry

- **Snack/Dessert:** Apple Cinnamon Walnut Muffins

Day 18:

- **Breakfast:** Turkey and Vegetable Breakfast Skewers

- **Lunch:** Cauliflower Rice and Shrimp Bowl

- **Dinner:** Stuffed Acorn Squash with Ground Bison

- **Snack/Dessert:** Pecan Pie Energy Bars

Day 19:

- **Breakfast:** Cauliflower and Broccoli Breakfast Casserole

- **Lunch:** Lentil and Vegetable Soup

- **Dinner:** Garlic Herb Roasted Chicken Thighs

- **Snack/Dessert:** Lemon Poppy Seed Coconut Flour Cookies

Day 20:

- **Breakfast:** Pesto and Tomato Breakfast Stuffed Avocado

- **Lunch:** Butternut Squash and Chicken Stew

- **Dinner:** Mushroom and Spinach Stuffed Chicken Breasts

- **Snack/Dessert:** Pumpkin Spice Pecan Cookies

Day 21:

- **Breakfast:** Lectin-Free Berry Smoothie Bowl

- **Lunch:** Grilled Chicken and Vegetable Salad

- **Dinner:** Baked Lemon Herb Chicken

- **Snack/Dessert:** Almond Butter Energy Bites

Day 22:

- **Breakfast:** Spinach and Tomato Omelette

- **Lunch:** Quinoa and Roasted Vegetable Bowl

- **Dinner:** Cauliflower Alfredo with Shrimp and Spinach

- **Snack/Dessert:** Chocolate Avocado Mousse

Day 23:

- **Breakfast:** Almond Flour Pancakes

- **Lunch:** Eggplant and Mushroom Stir-Fry

- **Dinner:** Turkey and Vegetable Stuffed Bell Peppers

- **Snack/Dessert:** Cinnamon Almond Roasted Chickpeas

Day 24:

- **Breakfast:** Avocado and Smoked Salmon Breakfast Wrap

- **Lunch:** Salmon and Asparagus Foil Packets

- **Dinner:** Eggplant Lasagna

- **Snack/Dessert:** Berry Chia Seed Pudding

Day 25:

- **Breakfast:** Chia Seed Pudding Parfait

- **Lunch:** Turkey and Vegetable Lettuce Wraps

- **Dinner:** Spaghetti Squash with Turkey Bolognese

- **Snack/Dessert:** Coconut Flour Banana Bread

Day 26:

- **Breakfast:** Sweet Potato and Kale Breakfast Hash

- **Lunch:** Cabbage and Chicken Stir-Fry

- **Dinner:** Lemon Garlic Shrimp and Broccoli Stir-Fry

- **Snack/Dessert:** Vanilla Almond Date Balls

Day 27:

- **Breakfast:** Turkey and Vegetable Breakfast Skewers

- **Lunch:** Cauliflower Rice and Shrimp Bowl

- **Dinner:** Stuffed Acorn Squash with Ground Bison

- **Snack/Dessert:** Pecan Pie Energy Bars

Day 28:

- **Breakfast:** Cauliflower and Broccoli Breakfast Casserole

- **Lunch:** Butternut Squash and Chicken Stew

- **Dinner:** Mushroom and Spinach Stuffed Chicken Breasts

- **Snack/Dessert:** Pumpkin Spice Pecan Cookies

CHAPTER 9: NAVIGATING SOCIAL SITUATIONS

Dining Out on a Lectin-Free Diet

Dining out can be a delightful experience, full of social interaction and delicious food. However, for those following a lectin-free diet, it can also present challenges. Navigating restaurant menus and ensuring your choices align with your dietary preferences requires a bit of strategic planning. Here's a guide on how to enjoy dining out while adhering to a lectin-free lifestyle.

Understanding Restaurant Menus: One of the first steps to successfully dining out on a lectin-free diet is to become familiar with common menu items and their potential lectin content. Dishes that often contain lectins include those with grains, legumes, and certain nightshade vegetables. Instead, focus on protein-rich options like grilled meats, fish, and poultry, along with a variety of non-starchy vegetables. Many restaurants also offer customizable salads, allowing you to choose lectin-free ingredients.

Researching Restaurants in Advance: Before heading to a restaurant, take advantage of online resources to research the menu. Many establishments now provide their menus on their websites, making it easier to plan ahead. Look for dishes that are likely to be lectin-free or can be modified to meet your requirements. If needed, don't hesitate to contact the restaurant directly to inquire about their ability to accommodate a lectin-free diet.

Communicating with the Waitstaff: Once you arrive at the restaurant, don't hesitate to communicate your dietary needs with the waitstaff. Be polite but clear about your restrictions, emphasizing the importance of avoiding certain ingredients. A friendly and open conversation can often lead to better understanding and a more enjoyable dining experience. Ask questions about the preparation methods and ingredients used in specific dishes to ensure they align with your lectin-free preferences.

Customizing Your Order: Many restaurants are willing to accommodate dietary preferences by allowing customization of dishes. For example, if a dish comes with a lectin-containing sauce, ask for it on the side or request a substitution. Similarly, if a menu item includes grains, inquire about the possibility of replacing them with a lectin-free alternative like extra vegetables or a side salad. Most establishments are willing to make adjustments to meet your dietary needs.

Choosing Safe Cuisine Types: Certain cuisines naturally lend themselves to lectin-free options. For instance, Mediterranean and Japanese cuisines often feature grilled proteins, fresh vegetables, and healthy fats. Italian restaurants may offer pasta alternatives like zucchini noodles or provide gluten-free options. By selecting restaurants that align with lectin-free-friendly cuisines, you increase your chances of finding suitable menu choices.

Communicating Your Dietary Needs

Effectively communicating your dietary needs is crucial, whether dining out with friends, attending social events, or simply sharing a meal at someone's home. Clear and respectful communication can help others understand your requirements and make the experience more enjoyable for everyone involved.

Educating Friends and Family: Those close to you may not be familiar with the intricacies of a lectin-free diet. Take the opportunity to educate friends and family about your dietary preferences. Share resources or guidelines that outline the foods you avoid and those you embrace. When planning gatherings, collaborate on menu options that accommodate both your dietary needs and the preferences of others.

Choosing Restaurants with Diverse Menus: When selecting restaurants for group outings, opt for establishments with diverse menus that cater to various dietary preferences. This can help ensure there are lectin-free options for you while offering a range of choices for your companions. Most restaurants strive to provide options for various dietary needs, making it easier to find something suitable for everyone.

Bringing a Dish to Share: If you're attending a social gathering or dinner party, consider bringing a lectin-free dish to share. Not only does this guarantee you'll have a safe option, but it also introduces others to delicious and nutritious lectin-free recipes. Sharing your culinary creations can spark interest and curiosity, fostering a positive environment around your dietary choices.

Using Positive Language: When discussing your dietary needs, use positive language to convey your preferences. Emphasize the foods you enjoy rather than focusing solely on restrictions. For example, instead of saying, "I can't eat bread," say, "I love incorporating a variety of vegetables into my meals." This approach helps frame the conversation in a positive light and may encourage others to be more accommodating.

Being Flexible and Grateful: While it's important to communicate your dietary needs, flexibility is also key. Not every social setting may provide perfect lectin-free options, and that's okay. Express gratitude for the efforts others make to accommodate your preferences, even if it means making small adjustments to your own plate. Being flexible and appreciative fosters positive relationships and makes social interactions more enjoyable for everyone.

CONCLUSION

As we wrap up our exploration of the lectin-free lifestyle, I hope you've found this journey insightful and practical. Navigating the intricacies of a lectin-free diet isn't just about eliminating certain foods; it's about embracing a new way of nourishing your body and enjoying a diverse range of delicious meals.

We started by delving into the fundamentals, understanding what lectins are and how they interact with our bodies. Armed with this knowledge, we ventured into the kitchen with comprehensive recipes for breakfast, lunch, dinner, and delightful snacks and desserts. These recipes weren't just about sustenance; they were crafted to be flavorful, satisfying, and easy to integrate into your daily life.

Chapters like "Getting Started with the Lectin-Free Diet" and "The Lectin-Free Kitchen" equipped you with practical tips, ensuring your pantry is stocked, your kitchen tools are ready, and your cooking techniques align with the lectin-free lifestyle. We explored the art of meal planning and prepping, making this transformative way of eating not just feasible but also efficient.

The journey extended beyond the confines of your kitchen and into the social sphere with "Navigating Social Situations." Dining out, communicating your dietary needs, and sharing your lectin-free journey with others are integral components of this lifestyle. It's about striking a balance between staying true to your principles and fostering positive connections with those around you.

Remember, the lectin-free lifestyle is not a rigid set of rules but a framework that empowers you to make informed choices about what you put on your plate. Flexibility is key, and so is the joy of discovery. Finding lectin-free options doesn't mean sacrificing flavor or variety; it opens the door to a world of vibrant, nutrient-rich foods waiting to be explored.

As you embark on this journey, celebrate the victories—whether it's mastering a new recipe, confidently ordering a lectin-free meal at a restaurant, or introducing loved ones to the delicious possibilities of this lifestyle. Embrace the learning process, and don't be too hard on yourself. Life is a continual journey of growth, and your approach to nutrition is a vital part of that evolution.

In closing, I encourage you to make this lectin-free lifestyle your own. Tweak the recipes, experiment with flavors, and listen to your body's signals. Whether you're drawn to the simplicity of a berry smoothie bowl, the comfort of a roasted vegetable bowl, or the elegance of a stuffed acorn squash, savor the journey.

Here's to your health, well-being, and the joy of discovering a lectin-free way of living—one delicious meal at a time. Cheers!